THE RIGHT WAY TO ACHIEVE A PERFECT BUILT

Top 10+ Essential Exercise To Burn Fat, Transform From being Lost And Unfit To Being Fit, Enjoying Physical Activities And Living Healthy

Dr. Lisa Blue

Contents

INTRODUCTION

An Overview Of The Significance Of Having A Well-Built Body

When starting the quest for the ideal build, a plethora of advice is frequently offered, which can leave many feeling confused and overwhelmed about where to begin. Let's examine a straightforward and practical strategy amid this confusion: "The Right Way to Achieve a Perfect Build."

This is a simple manual that concentrates on fundamental ideas rather than intricate equations or drastic methods. Think of it as a compass that will lead you to your fitness objectives in a sustainable and balanced manner.

Starting this journey starts with understanding your body. It's important to acknowledge your talents and areas for growth rather than comparing yourself to other people. In this straightforward story, we'll examine how gradual, little modifications can result in big advancements.

A key component of every fitness regimen, nutrition doesn't have to be complicated. Here, the emphasis is on making deliberate decisions and adopting a diet that feeds your body without needless limitations. Think of this as a slow transition to a better relationship with food, where every decision you make improves your general health.

Exercise doesn't have to be a difficult math problem either. Consider it instead as a sequence of happy and aligning movements. Simplicity is key, whether you're doing weightlifting, dancing, or fast walking. The approach that works best for you is the one that makes working out a fun and sustainable part of your everyday life.

This is a journey of gradual growth rather than a sprint. There's no need to make significant life-altering adjustments or take severe actions. When combined, small, steady steps make up a tapestry of progress. After all, it's progress, not perfection, that matters.

According to "The Right Way to Achieve a Perfect Build," simplicity takes center stage. It's an offer to accept a simple yet effective route to becoming a fitter, healthier version of yourself.

Welcome to **"The Right Way to Achieve a Perfect Build,"** a tutorial that communicates in terms of ease of use. Here, we simplify the confusing world of fitness and provide an easy-to-follow path to your objectives. It's an invitation to embark on a journey that will lead to a balanced, healthier version of yourself rather than some far-off ideal.

CHAPTER ONE

Realistic Expectations and Goals

Whether it's for personal growth, career advancement, or health, the foundation of any successful journey is setting reasonable expectations and goals. It's like laying out a route to get somewhere; the more precise the map, the easier the trip will be.

A realistic aim fits your current situation and skill level. These are attainable benchmarks that help you advance, not dreams. Setting achievable goals is beautiful because it encourages growth without leading to dissatisfaction.

Conversely, expectations are the sentimental relatives of aims. They are the expectations, the imagined schematics of the possible course of the adventure. Recognizing that growth isn't necessarily linear and that there may be peaks and valleys, detours, and breathtaking views is necessary to set reasonable expectations.

Why is that so important? Because disappointment and exhaustion frequently arise from the discrepancy between expectations and reality. Imagine starting a fitness adventure to consistently improve quickly. The truth may include lulls in the action, exhausting times, or sporadic setbacks. But when one has reasonable expectations, these don't seem like insurmountable obstacles; rather, they blend in with the surroundings.

Achievable objectives serve as markers to help you stay on track. If you've never run a marathon, set a goal like running a 5K in three months instead of trying to complete a marathon in less than a month. SMART stands for specified, measurable, achievable, relevant, and time-bound; it is the formula for creating feasible objectives.

In a similar vein, reasonable expectations reduce the emotional strain. If losing weight is your aim, be aware that healthy weight reduction happens gradually. Having unrealistic expectations might lead to disappointment because it may entail expecting significant improvements overnight.

Flexibility is also another essential component. Because life is unpredictable, things might change. A more sustainable and flexible path is made possible by having an open mind to change as circumstances demand that you modify your expectations and ambitions.

Finding a balance between pushing yourself and realizing your current limitations is the essence of having reasonable expectations and goals. It's about cultivating an attitude that values the process just as much as the result and recognizes any progress, no matter how tiny.

So, consider your goals for a moment, whether they are related to personal development, job aspirations, or physical accomplishments. Are they attainable in your present situation? Do they permit adaptability and self-empathy? When you lower your expectations appropriately, the path becomes not only feasible but also incredibly fulfilling.

Knowing Your Body

The essential step to opening the door to personal well-being is understanding your body. It's similar to having the owner's manual for a sophisticated, well-tuned machine—your body. The greater your understanding of its responses, features, and particularities, the more capable you will be of making choices that advance your general health and well-being.

The first step in this self-discovery journey is to accept the uniqueness of your body. Everybody's body is different, reacting differently to diverse stimuli, just as no two fingerprints are alike. The basis of this awareness is realizing your body's unique demands, capabilities, and weaknesses.

Think about your body type: Are you an endomorph, mesomorph, or ectomorph? This classification is about knowing how your body responds to exercise and nutrition, not about trying to fit into a preconceived model. It's a place to start when you customize your wellness strategy to fit your body's innate patterns.

Understanding the subtle messages your body sends is just as important as listening to them. Your body sends signals through hunger, thirst, weariness, and even mood swings. Understanding how to interpret these cues enables you to customize your lifestyle, including your nutrition, exercise regimen, and when and how much rest to get.

Recognizing the effects of outside influences is another aspect of understanding your body. Factors such as sleep patterns, stress levels, lifestyle decisions, and environmental factors can all impact your general health. You can use this awareness to make deliberate decisions that improve the balance of your body.

Think about your body's amazing systems as you explore its nuances: the neurological, musculoskeletal, and cardiovascular systems all function in perfect harmony. Understanding the distinct roles that each system plays will help you customize your exercise regimen to improve your general health.

Understanding how your body metabolizes various nutrients is crucial when it comes to nutrition. Do you find that a well-balanced macronutrient consumption suits you better than a larger protein intake? With this knowledge, you may design a diet that keeps you motivated and helps you reach your objectives.

The goal of this body-awareness journey is not instant mastery or perfection. It's an ongoing process of discovery and collaboration with your own body. The more knowledge you acquire, the more capable you are of making decisions that are in sync with the rhythm of your own body.

Knowing your body is, at its core, a journey of self-awareness. It's about having a loving conversation with your body and accepting it as a dynamic, always-changing creature. This information is a compass that leads you on a path to a happier, better life; it is more than just power.

Body Types And How They Affect Exercise

Knowing your body type will help you create a training plan that is both efficient and unique to you. Ectomorph, mesomorph, and endomorph are the three main body types. Each has certain traits that affect how people react to exercise, diet, and fitness regimens in general.

- **Ectomorph**

Features: Ectomorphs are usually described as having a slim, lean body with narrow hips and shoulders. They frequently have quick metabolisms, which makes it difficult for them to put on weight and grow muscle.

Effect on Training: Ectomorphs may have trouble gaining muscle bulk, yet they usually thrive in endurance sports. To promote muscle growth, their training should emphasize complex exercises combined with progressive resistance training. To promote muscle growth, a balanced macronutrient ratio and an adequate calorie intake are also essential.

- **Mesomorph**

Features: Mesomorphs have a wider shoulder-to-hip ratio and are inherently muscular and well-proportioned. They typically lose fat and increase muscle quickly.

Effect on Training: Mesomorphs frequently react favorably to a range of training strategies. They can perform both isolation and complex exercises as part of a strength and resistance training program. It's crucial to keep a balanced diet, with a focus on protein consumption for the upkeep and development of muscle.

- **Endomorph**

Features: Endomorphs tend to be rounder, softer, and more likely to accumulate fat on their bodies.

They might have a slower metabolism, which would facilitate weight gain.

Impact on Training: Endomorphs gain from a training regimen that mixes resistance training and cardiovascular exercise. This mixture increases lean muscle mass and aids in the management of body fat. For burning calories, high-intensity interval training (HIIT) can be especially beneficial. To assist weight management, nutrition is important, with a focus on portion control and a balanced diet.

It's crucial to remember that these body types are not fixed, and many people may have traits of more than one kind. In addition, a person's lifestyle, genetics, and age all have a big impact on their physical characteristics.

In the end, it all comes down to customizing your workout regimen to fit your body type and objectives. It's critical to regularly analyze your body and make adjustments based on how it responds to training. Speaking with a healthcare provider or fitness expert might help you receive more advice that is unique to your goals and needs.

CHAPTER TWO

Evaluating Your Level Of Fitness Right Now

Evaluating your current level of fitness is an essential first step in achieving better health and well-being. It gives you a baseline awareness of your physical condition, capabilities, and weaknesses, enabling you to create a fitness program that suits your needs and establishes realistic goals. *When assessing your present level of fitness, keep the following important factors in mind:*

Heart-Related Endurance:
•Evaluate your endurance for prolonged periods of aerobic exercise. This could involve exercises like swimming, cycling, jogging, or walking.

•To measure your cardiovascular fitness, try the 1-mile walk or run, the 3-minute step test, or the 12-minute run.

Muscular Power:

•Use workouts that focus on your main muscle groups to assess your level of muscle strength. Push-ups are a common test for upper body strength, and lunges or squats are a common test for lower body strength.

•Take into consideration measuring your maximal strength during different exercises using weights or resistance bands.

Physique Endurance:

•Your muscles' capacity for prolonged, repetitive motion is measured by muscular endurance. Exercises like plank hold, bodyweight squats, and tricep dips can be used to gauge this.

•Find out how many reps you can do with good form before you start to feel tired.

Adaptability

•Maintaining joint health and preventing injuries need flexibility. Use stretches for your shoulders, yoga positions, or the sit-and-reach test to gauge your level of flexibility.

•To find out how flexible you are, make a note of how far you can stretch in different directions without discomfort.

physique composition

•Knowing your body's composition, which includes the proportion of muscle to fat, can tell you a lot about your general health. Dual-energy X-ray absorptiometry **(DEXA)** scans, skinfold caliper measures, and bioelectrical impedance analysis **(BIA)** are common techniques.

•It might be more beneficial to monitor changes in your body composition over time as opposed to just your weight.

Stability and Equilibrium:

•Evaluating your stability and balance is essential for general functional fitness. Your stability can be assessed using easy activities like standing on one leg or balancing on an uneven surface.

•Observe how well you can stay balanced while performing different tasks.

Flexibility and Sync:

•Activities that call for rapid, precise movements demand coordination and agility. Exercises like ladder drills, cone drills, or movements particular to your sport can help you gauge your agility.

•To assess your agility and coordination, pay close attention to the speed and accuracy of your movements.

Recall that the purpose of evaluating your level of fitness is to establish a unique beginning point for your fitness journey rather than to measure yourself against others. Knowing where you stand will help you set realistic objectives and gradually increase your level of fitness over time.

Before Beginning A Fitness Adventure, Consider Your Health

Starting a fitness journey is a great decision, but before getting started, it's important to consider several health factors. Making sure your body is prepared for more exercise is essential to achieving a long-term, safe fitness goal. The following are important health factors to remember:

- **Health History:**

✓Consult a healthcare provider to go over your medical history to determine whether any current ailments, long-term illnesses, or past injuries may affect your capacity to perform specific workouts.

✓Talk to your doctor about any medications you take, as some may affect how you exercise.

- **Previous Health Issues:**

✓See your healthcare practitioner to find out what kind and level of exercise is safe for you if you have any pre-existing diseases, such as respiratory, orthopedic, diabetic, or cardiovascular problems.

✓A fitness program under medical supervision may be beneficial for people with long-term medical issues.

- **Physical Fitness Evaluation:**

✓To determine your current level of fitness, perform a fitness assessment or speak with a fitness specialist. This aids in creating a program that suits your skills and objectives.

✓Measurements of body composition, physical strength, flexibility, and cardiovascular endurance are a few examples of assessments.

- **Movement and Joint Health:**

✓Assess the mobility and health of your joints, particularly if you have arthritis or other joint-related conditions. It may be more appropriate to engage in low-impact activities like swimming, cycling, or elliptical training.

✓To increase joint flexibility and lower your chance of injury, include stretches and mobility exercises in your routine.

- **Age and Degree of Fitness:**

✓As you arrange your exercise regimen, take into account your age and present level of fitness. Exercises that emphasize strength, flexibility, and balance can help older persons maintain their general health.

✓Beginners should begin cautiously so that the body can gradually adjust to higher levels of activity.

- **Expectancy:**

✓Before beginning or altering an exercise regimen while pregnant, speak with your healthcare physician. While exercising safely while pregnant might improve general health, there may be some things to watch out for.

✓Choose low-impact pursuits over strenuous workouts that strain the abdomen region excessively.

- **Dietary considerations**

✓Make sure you're giving your body the right kind of fuel by eating a healthy, balanced diet. Healthy eating maintains your energy levels, promotes healing, and amplifies the advantages of your exercise endeavors.

✓Drink plenty of water, especially when working out, to promote maximum efficiency and recuperation.

- **Consultation with Exercise Specialists**

✓Consult a licensed fitness professional for advice if you're unclear on where to begin or how to organize your workout routine. They can offer tailored guidance depending on your objectives and current state of health.

Recall that putting your health first and taking a holistic approach is the key to a successful fitness journey. You can design a safe and efficient plan that puts you on the road to better fitness and general health by taking these health aspects into account.

CHAPTER THREE

Laying The Groundwork: Diet

Establishing a strong nutritional base is critical to maintaining general health, energy levels, and peak performance on any fitness journey. When creating this nutritious basis, keep the following important points in mind:

Healthy Diet:

•A well-balanced diet should consist of a range of whole foods from every dietary group. This guarantees a wide variety of nutrients, such as lipids, proteins, carbs, vitamins, and minerals.

•Eat a variety of complex carbs (whole grains, fruits, and vegetables), lean proteins (chicken, fish, and legumes), and healthy fats (nuts, seeds, and avocados) with your meals.

Control of Portion:

•To avoid overindulging and to keep your weight within a healthy range, practice portion management. Consider portion sizes and pay attention to your body's signals of hunger and fullness.

•To assist in controlling portion sizes, use smaller bowls and plates, and steer clear of ingesting a lot of high-calorie, low-nutrient items.

Hydration

•To stay well hydrated all day, sip water.

•Water is necessary for several body processes, such as temperature regulation, nutrition absorption, and digestion.

Reduce your consumption of sugar-filled drinks and make water your main source of hydration.

Meal Schedule:

•To promote energy levels and healing, think about when to eat and when to snack. Consistent energy levels can be achieved by eating smaller, more balanced meals every three to four hours.

•Eat a well-balanced supper or snack that includes both protein and carbs before and after working out if you're exercising.

Vitamin Timing:

•Be mindful of when to take certain nutrients, particularly when working on exercise.
•Energy can be obtained by consuming a combination of carbs and protein before exercise, glycogen stores are replenished and muscle repair is supported by a post-workout meal.

Conscious Eating:

•Eat mindfully by focusing solely on your food and avoiding outside distractions. To avoid overindulging, take pleasure in your meal and pay attention to your body's cues of hunger and fullness.

•Take gaps between bites to allow your body to register fullness, and chew and taste your food to the fullest.

Eat Fewer Processed Foods:

•Reduce your consumption of refined and highly processed foods, which frequently include additional sugars, bad fats, and fewer nutrients. For best health, concentrate on eating full, nutrient-dense foods.

•Pay attention to ingredient lists and food labels, and select products with the fewest additives and preservatives possible.

Personalized Method

•Understand that each person has different nutritional demands depending on their age, gender, degree of exercise, and overall health. •To customize your nutrition plan to your unique requirements and objectives, think about speaking with a registered dietitian or other nutrition specialist.

Continuity:

•When constructing a dietary basis, consistency is essential. Gradually developing good eating habits promotes improved digestion, long-term energy, and general health.

•To help your fitness journey, stay away from excessive diets and concentrate on making long-term, sustainable adjustments.

•You'll create a strong foundation that supports general health and your fitness objectives by implementing these ideas into your nutritional strategy.

The Value of Of A Well-Balanced Diet

The foundation of general health and well-being is a balanced diet. It gives the body the nutrition it needs, such as proteins for healing tissue, fats for energy, and a variety of vitamins and minerals for healthy physiological processes. A balanced diet lowers the chance of developing chronic illnesses while promoting healthy growth, development, and immune system performance. It guarantees that the body gets the proper ratios of nutrients, promoting a balanced interaction that maintains both mental and physical well-being. A balanced diet also supports healthy digestion, blood sugar regulation, and maintaining a healthy weight. A balanced diet is essential to a long life and a healthy, active lifestyle because it provides the body with a range of nutrients in the right amounts.

Furthermore, a healthy diet influences mood and cognitive function, both of which are important for mental health. Foods high in nutrients, like fruits, vegetables, and whole grains, include antioxidants that promote mental wellness. Eating a healthy diet has been associated with enhanced mental toughness, memory, and focus. A balanced diet helps to stabilize blood sugar levels, which helps to minimize fatigue and energy dips and maintain steady energy levels throughout the day.

Beyond its advantages, a balanced diet is essential for managing and preventing several illnesses, such as diabetes, obesity, and cardiovascular diseases. It promotes a healthy relationship with food by highlighting the value of variety and moderation. In the end, a balanced diet is a comprehensive strategy for nourishing the body and mind, fostering vigor, and creating the groundwork for a longer, healthier life. It goes beyond simply providing for basic needs.

The Functions Of Macronutrients (proteins, carbs, and fats)

The key nutrients known as macronutrients are needed by the body in comparatively high quantities to provide the energy needed for daily activities. The three basic macronutrients are lipids, proteins, and carbohydrates. Each has a unique function in preserving general health.

- **The protein**

Function: Proteins are the body's building blocks and are essential for tissue growth, maintenance, and repair. Enzymes, hormones, and immune system components are all synthesized by them.

Sources: Dairy products, eggs, meat, poultry, fish, legumes, nuts, and seeds.

-

Function: The body uses carbohydrates as its main energy source. They are converted into glucose, which powers several body processes, most notably mental and physical activity.

Whole grains, veggies, fruits, legumes, and starchy foods like potatoes are some of the **sources.**

-

Function: Fats provide a concentrated source of energy and are necessary for the absorption of vitamins that are soluble in fat **(A, D, E, and K).** They aid in the manufacturing of hormones and assist in the insulation and structure of cells.

Sources: Nuts, seeds, avocados, olive oil, and fatty fish are good sources of healthy fats. Limit the amount of processed food's saturated and trans fats.

Maintaining a well-rounded diet requires balancing the intake of various macronutrients. Depending on personal objectives, exercise levels, and general health, the ratios of each macronutrient may change. A well-balanced mixture promotes many elements of health, from immune system function to energy metabolism, and guarantees the body gets the nutrients it needs to perform at its best.

CHAPTER FOUR

Exercises Of The Cardiovascular System

Swimming

Is easy on the joints and works with a variety of muscle groups.

Immerse yourself in the revitalizing sport of swimming, which is a lively, low-impact workout with many advantages.

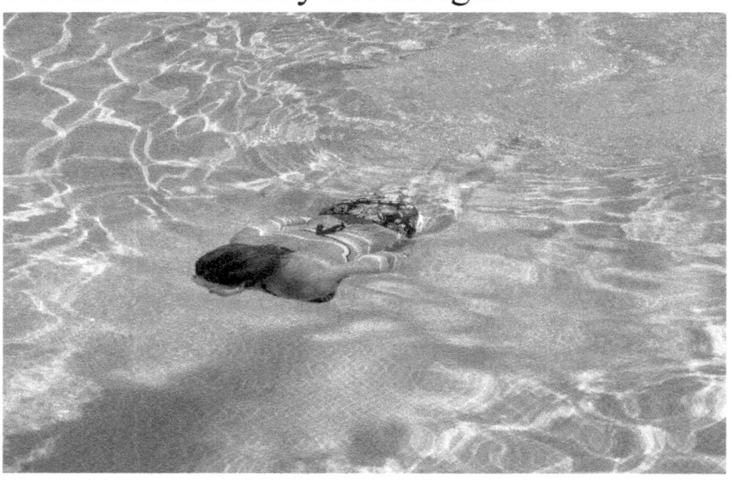

Step 1: Prepare

Make sure you have the necessities: a swim cap, goggles, and well-fitting swimwear. These fundamentals guarantee your comfort and improve your swimming experience.

Step 2: Select Your Artery

Choose a swimming stroke based on your comfort level and fitness objectives. Every stroke works a different set of muscles, whether it's the forceful butterfly, the soothing backstroke, or the freestyle for a full-body workout.

Step 3: Get Ready

Warm up for a little while before starting the main set. To improve circulation, release tension in your muscles, and get your body ready for more strenuous exercise, swim a few laps at a leisurely pace.

Step 4: Create a Schedule

Create a swimming regimen that supports your fitness goals. Consistency is essential, whether you're doing an interval training program for cardiovascular health or a leisurely swim to relieve stress.

Step 5: Pay Attention to Methods

Put using the right method first to get the most out of it and avoid being hurt. Seek the advice of a swim instructor or make use of internet resources to improve your breathing and stroke technique.

Step 6: Steady Advancement

Gradually increase the length and intensity of your swims as your confidence grows. Reaching fitness goals and continuing to improve require progression.

Swimming is a complete workout that works the body and the mind, in addition to being a cool retreat. Jump in, create a splash, and discover all of the advantages of this adaptable and restorative workout.

Jogging/Running

Jogging or running is a time-tested and efficient method of burning calories.

Take up the thrilling sport of running or jogging, which is a multipurpose cardiovascular exercise that enhances both physical and mental health.

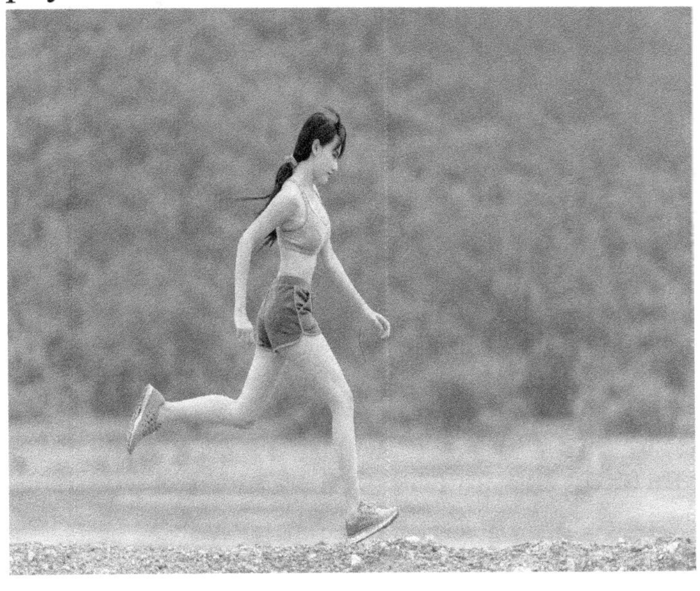

Step 1: Adequate Footwear

Invest in supportive, cushioned, and properly fitting running shoes. Wearing the proper shoes guarantees comfort and reduces the risk of repetitive impact injuries.

Step 2: Daily Warm-Up

Warming up at the start of your run will help your muscles and joints become ready for the exercise. You can increase your heart rate and increase your flexibility by doing dynamic stretches, light running, or quick walking for a short while.

Step 3: Select an Appropriate Surface

Choose a running surface based on how comfortable and fit you are. Choosing the correct terrain may affect your entire experience, whether it's the cushioned track of a field, the steady concrete of a road, or the forgiving surface of a trail.

Step Four: Steady Advancement

Begin at a speed appropriate for your present level of fitness and increase distance and intensity gradually. By taking it gradually, you lower your chance of overuse problems and give your body time to adjust to the demands of running.

Step 5: Give Form Priority

Sustain good running form to maximize performance and lower your chance of injury. For a fluid and controlled run, pay attention to your arm movement, posture, and stride length.

Step 6: Blend It

Add diversity to your jogging regimen to keep it interesting. To make your workouts more exciting and challenging, try trail running, interval training, or joining a running group.

Step 7: Rest and Recuperation

Make healing your priority by scheduling rest days into your schedule. Sufficient sleep facilitates physical recovery, averts burnout, and encourages sustained endurance in your running endeavors.

Running and jogging provide an engaging and approachable route to fitness, regardless of your goals—relief from stress, weight control, or enhanced cardiovascular health. Put on your running shoes, hit the road, and enjoy the energizing effects of this age-old and powerful workout.

Cycling

Cycling Increases flexibility and uses the entire core.

Set off on a cycling adventure: a fun and adaptable workout that combines the excitement of discovery with cardiovascular benefits.

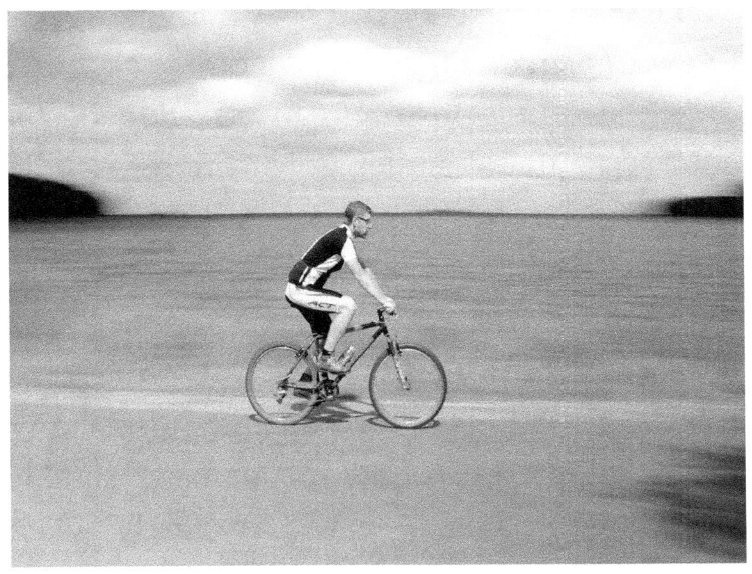

Step 1: Pick the Correct Bicycle

Choose a bike based on its intended purpose. While mountain bikes are designed for rough terrain, road bikes are best for speed and distance. Bicycles with hybrid technology offer a flexible choice for various terrains.

Step 2: Suitable Bike Fit

Make sure your bike fits your body correctly to avoid pain and damage. A comfortable and effective riding position can be achieved by adjusting the handlebar position, saddle height, and overall bike geometry.

Step3: Prioritize safety

Put safety first by using a helmet and observing traffic laws. Make sure your bike has the right lights and reflectors, especially in low light. Learn how to use hand signals so that you can communicate clearly when driving.

Step 4: Begin with brief excursions

Start with short rides to gain confidence and familiarize yourself with your bike. As your fitness improves, gradually increase the length and intensity of your rides.

Step 5: Examine Various Paths

To keep your cycling experience exciting, try out different routes. Adding variety to your rides increases mental and physical stimulation, whether you want to cycle on tough hills, picturesque trails, or through metropolitan environments.

Step 6: Include Recurring Instruction

Increase cardiovascular fitness and burn calories by including interval training in your cycling regimen. For a dynamic workout, alternate between high-intensity and rest intervals.

Step 7: Upkeep Inspections

Check for wear and tear on your bike regularly. To improve performance and safety, oil the chain, check the tire pressure, and make sure the brakes and gears are working properly.

Cycling offers a low-impact, friendly-to-joint cardiovascular workout in addition to opening doors to new experiences. Cycling offers a personalized fitness journey that suits all skill levels, from easy rides to strenuous peaks. Put on your saddlebags, feel the breeze on your face, and pedal in the direction of a more energetic, healthful living.

Rowing

Take up rowing for a full-body workout; it's a low-impact, high-efficiency activity that works for several muscle groups and improves cardiovascular health.

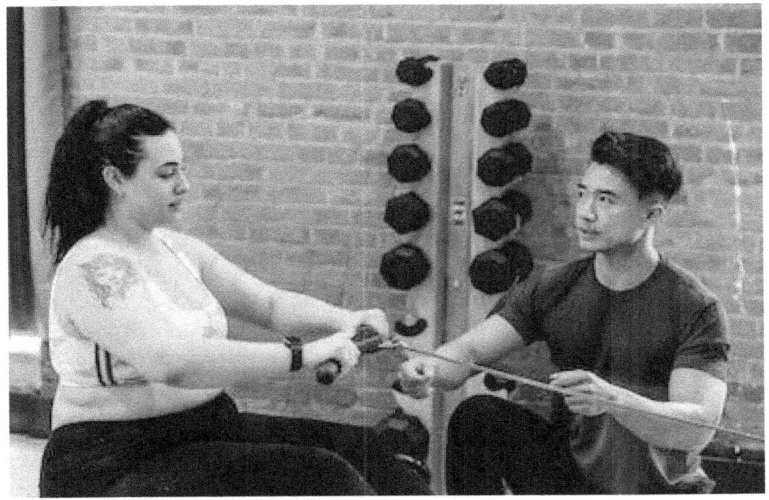

Step1: Use the Right Method

It's critical to acquire the proper rowing technique. To enhance each stroke's efficacy, make sure your posture is correct and your arm movements are coordinated with your leg drive.

Step 2: Configuring the Rowing Device

Configure the rowing machine according to your needs. For a customized and pleasant experience, place your feet in the foot straps, adjust the difficulty level, and become acquainted with the machine's settings.

Step 3: Get Ready

Warm up before starting your rowing exercise by doing some mild rowing at a comfortable pace. Your muscles and joints get ready for the upcoming, more strenuous workout.

Step 4: Pay Attention to Stroke Rate

Track your stroke rate while maintaining a power-to-speed ratio. By maintaining a steady and effective stroke rate, you can make the most of every rowing effort.

Step 6: Gradual Intensity

As your fitness level increases, start with a modest effort and progressively increase the resistance or time. Easy development is possible with rowing since it doesn't have the same impact as some other activities.

Step 6: Training Intervals

To make your rowing program more interesting and challenging, include interval training. A combination of high-intensity rowing and active recovery intervals increases calorie burn and cardiovascular fitness.

Step 7: Stretching and Cooling Down

Stretching comes after your rowing exercise, and then cool-down. This increases general recuperation, eases soreness in the muscles, and encourages flexibility.

An effective full-body workout that simultaneously works the muscles in the upper, core, and legs is provided by rowing. The repetitive motion of rowing provides an excellent, low-impact workout that can be done by people of all fitness levels. Take advantage of every stroke, embrace the rowing machine, and row your way to a healthier, stronger version of yourself.

Rope Jump

With the help of jump rope, you may start a dynamic and efficient cardiovascular workout. This age-old activity promotes coordination, agility, and endurance in addition to cardiovascular fitness.

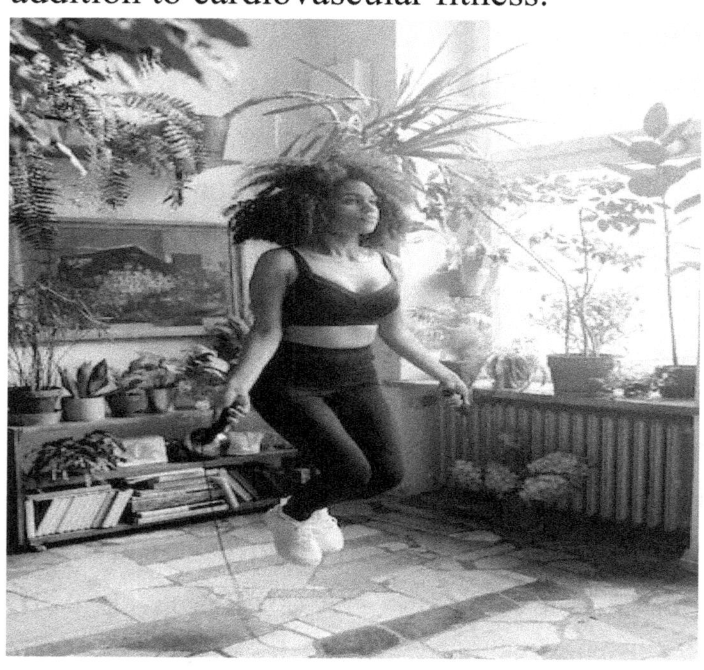

Step1: Choose the Correct Jump Rope

Select a jump rope based on your training objectives and degree of fitness. Beginners should use a simple PVC or beaded rope; experienced users can use a speed rope to rotate more quickly.

Step2: Correct Form

To enhance efficacy and reduce the chance of damage, maintain good form. Jump with a slight bend in your knees and the balls of your feet while maintaining your elbows close to your body and your wrists relaxed.

Step 3: Begin with simple leaps

Start with simple leaps to develop your coordination and rhythm. Pay close attention to when you jump and how smoothly the rope rotates. Try out some variants as you get better, including high knees or single-leg jumps.

Step 4: Gradual Intensity

By using interval training, you can progressively raise the intensity. Slower recuperation jumps and higher-intensity, faster-paced jumps should be alternated. This improves cardiovascular fitness and calorie burn.

Step 5: Diverse Methods

Try out some different jump rope moves, like side swings, crisscrosses, and double-unders (two revolutions every leap). These modifications not only make exercises interesting but also focus on various muscle groups.

Step 6: Progress and Consistency

The key is consistency. Include jump rope workouts regularly. As your fitness level increases, you can increase the length or intensity of the exercises. It's an easy workout to remain on schedule because it's portable and adaptable, and you can perform it anywhere.

Step 7: Stretching and Cooling Down

Finish your jump rope workout with a quick stretch and cool-down. This improves flexibility and helps avoid tense muscles.

Jump rope is an effective and easily accessible workout suitable for all levels of fitness. Jumping rope is a simple and adaptable exercise that can increase heart rate, burn calories, and help you develop a leaner, more agile body. Seize a rope, establish a rhythm, and launch yourself into a productive workout.

CHAPTER FIVE

Exercises For Strength Training

Squats: Engage your legs' major muscles

Work the back and legs as well as other major muscle groups.

Learn how to maximize the benefits of squats, a vital compound exercise that works the quadriceps, hamstrings, glutes, and core. To get the most out of your squats and avoid injuries, you must learn perfect form.

Step1: adopt a stance.

Place your toes slightly outward and place your feet shoulder-width apart or somewhat wider. The squat exercise has a solid base thanks to this stance.

Step 2: Contract Your Core Muscles

To keep your spine stable, brace your core muscles. This improves general balance and control while safeguarding your lower back.

Step 3: Set Off the Fall

Hinge at the hips and bend your knees to begin the squat. Throughout the exercise, keep your spine neutral and your chest elevated

Step 4: Bring Your Body Down

As though you were reclining in an imaginary chair, lower your body. Make sure your knees pass over your toes as you attempt to lower your thighs to parallelism.

Step 5: Preserve the Correct Form

Make sure your knees are parallel to your feet and do not allow them to buckle inward. To equally distribute the weight across your feet, maintain your weight on your heels.

Step 6: Use Power to Ascend

To get out of the squat, press through your heels. To properly engage the hip muscles, squeeze your glutes at the apex of the action.

Step 7: Continue and Advance

For the required number of repetitions, perform the squat motion again. As your strength increases, progressively increase the resistance by using weights, or switch up your squat technique by doing front squats or goblet squats.

Squats are a great way to increase lower body strength and improve overall functional fitness in your training program. Pay attention to form, raise the difficulty level gradually, and experience the life-changing power of this basic exercise.

Lunges: Work the legs and enhance stability and balance.

Lunges are a great compound exercise to add intensity to your leg-day program since they improve stability and balance while working the quads, hamstrings, glutes, and calves.

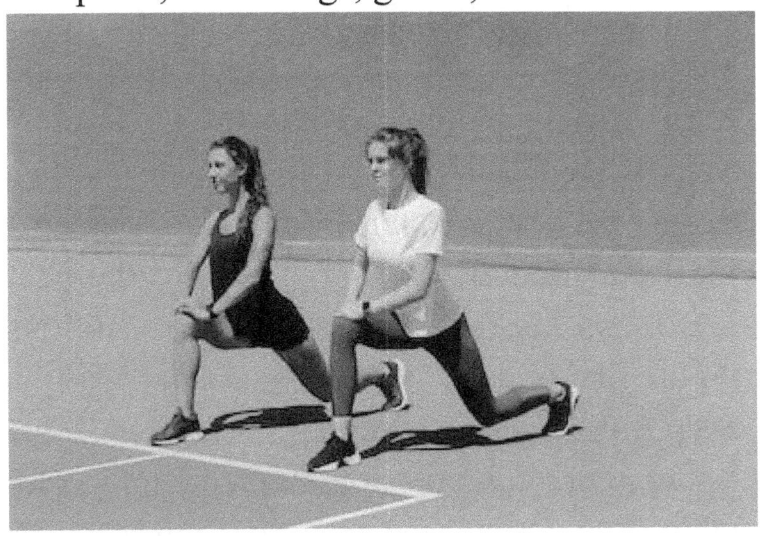

Step 1: Take a Tall stance.

Start by putting your feet hip-width apart and standing tall. Keep your body in alignment and use your core for support.

Step 2: Move In Front

Step forward with one foot, making sure your stride is long enough for both knees to bend 90 degrees when you lower yourself.

Step 3: Bring Your Body Down

Bend both of your knees to lower your body, making sure the back knee is just above the floor and the front knee is precisely over your ankle. Remain upright in your torso and refrain from bending forward.

Step 4: Rebound

To get back to the starting position, push off the front foot. Before moving on to the next leg, finish the required amount of repetitions on the first one.

Step 5: Lunges in reverse

As an alternative, try doing reverse lunges by taking steps backward as opposed to forward. This version is kinder to the knees and uses the muscles differently.

Step 6: Lunges Laterally

Step aside to incorporate lateral lunges. This adds variation to your workout by focusing on the inner and outer thighs.

Step 7: Advancement and Regularity

For a dynamic challenge, try including walking lunges or increasing the resistance as your strength increases.

Maintaining consistency is essential for optimizing the advantages of lunges, strengthening the lower body, and boosting functional fitness.

Push-ups: Target the core, triceps, shoulders, and chest.

A basic bodyweight exercise that works the triceps, shoulders, core, and chest well is the push-up. Acquiring proficiency in the correct form guarantees maximum activation of muscle groups and mitigates tension. *For successful push-ups, adhere to these steps:*

Step 1. Beginning Point:
Start in the plank position with your hands slightly wider than shoulder-width apart.
Step 2. Physical Alignment:
From head to heels, keep your body in a straight line and engage your core for stability.
Step 3. Hand Positioning:
With your fingers pointed forward or slightly outward, place your hands beneath your shoulders.

Step 4. Elbow Alignment

Keep your elbows close to your sides as you stoop to lower yourself toward the ground.

5. Darkness

Lower your chest as low as your strength will allow, or just over the floor.

Step 6. Full Range of Motion:

To reach the complete range of motion, extend your arms fully at the top of the exercise.

Step 7. Inhalation

Breathe in as you descend and exhale as you ascend again.

Step 8. Central Activation:

Keep your core strong to maintain stability during the exercise.

Step 9. Head Position:

To avoid putting too much tension on your neck, keep your head neutral and your eyes slightly forward.

10. Foot Alignment:
- Keep your feet hip-width apart or together, depending on your comfort and stability.

In addition to strengthening your upper body, push-ups also help to increase your core stability and overall functional fitness. This versatile exercise requires regular practice with proper form in order to reap its full benefits.

Exercise the upper body, particularly the back and biceps, with pull-ups and chin-ups.

Pull-ups and chin-ups are two challenging exercises that strengthen your upper body while targeting your shoulders, biceps, and back. Having proper form is essential to carrying out a work in a safe and efficient manner. To execute a strong pull-up or chin-up, do the following:

Step 1. Pause:

When doing pull-ups, use an overhand hold with your hands facing away from you. For chin-ups, use an underhand grip and point your hands in your direction.

Step 2. Hand Position:

Your hands should be placed slightly wider than shoulder-width apart for pull-ups and closer for chin-ups.

Step 3. Hanging Position:

Hang from the bar with your arms fully stretched and your shoulder blades clenched.

Step 4. Central Activation:

Contract your core muscles to maintain a straight posture.

Step 5. Making the Motion Start:

To begin the pull, flex your shoulder blades together and shift your torso toward the bar.

Step 6. Full Range of Motion:

Bring your chest to the bar for chin-ups and your chin over it for pull-ups. Achieve a complete range of motion.

Step 7. Consistent Drop:

Lower your body slowly and extend your arms fully before starting the next repetition.

Step 8. Breathing:

As you lift yourself up, exhale, and as you lower yourself back down, breathe in.

9. Gradual Progression:

If you're just getting started, start with assisted pull-ups or chin-ups and progressively reduce the assistance as your strength grows.

10. Consistency:

Pull-ups and chin-ups are great exercises to incorporate into your routine to build upper body strength gradually.

In addition to increasing muscle mass, compound workouts like pull-ups and chin-ups also enhance functional fitness. Regardless of your objective—stronger or more developed muscles—these exercises offer a demanding but rewarding upper-body session.

CHAPTER SIX

Exercises For Bodyweight Training

Burpees: This exercise blends strength and cardio.

Burpees combine strength training, cardio, and agility into an intensive, full-body exercise. Due to its ability to target many muscle groups and elevate heart rate, this is an excellent method for enhancing the intensity of any workout program.

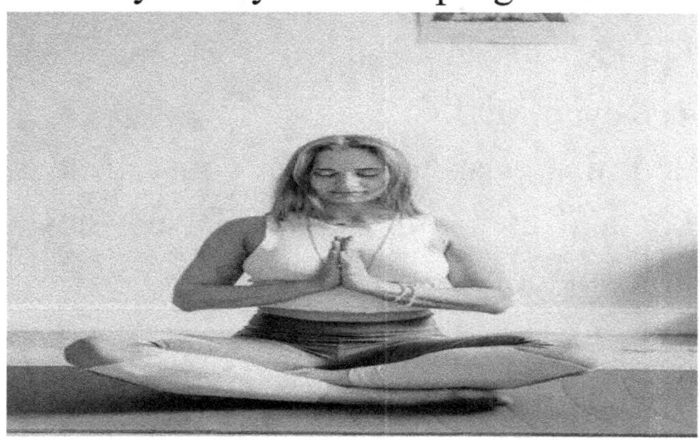

To execute a flawless burpee, adhere to these guidelines:

Step 1. Point of origin:

Place your feet shoulder-width apart as you enter the stage.

Step 2. Squat Down:

To lower yourself into a squat, bend your knees and place your hands on the floor in front of you.

Step 3. Inverted Leap:

Take a backward leap with your feet and land in a plank position.

From head to heels, your body should be in a straight line.

Step 4. Reversal:

To perform a push-up, lower your chest to the floor and then raise yourself back up to the plank position.

Step 5. Launch:

Leap your feet back toward your hands to return to a squat.

Step 6. Exploding Jump:

With a powerful lunge forward, lift your arms above your head.

Step 7. Repeat:

Land and immediately begin the next repetition.

Step 8. Breathing:

Breathe in during planking and squats and out during push-ups and leaps.

Step 9. Modification:

Adjust to your level of fitness by reducing the effort or missing the push-ups.

Burpees are a great exercise routine to improve overall strength and agility, cardiovascular fitness, and endurance. Adjust the intensity to your current level of fitness and enjoy all the benefits of this tough yet effective workout.

Mountain Climbers: Develops the core, legs, and shoulders.

Mountain climbers are a vigorous and efficient exercise that tones your arms, legs, and core while raising your heart rate. Including mountain climbers into your workout routine enhances your overall stamina, agility, and coordination. To guarantee effective implementation, adhere to these steps:

Step 1. Point of origin:

Assume the plank posture, placing your hands just below your shoulders and your torso in a straight line from your head to your heels.

Step 2. Principal Concern:

Contract your core muscles to maintain your body's stability and support your lower back.

Step 3. Press Knee Towards Chest:

As you bring your right leg up toward your chest, make sure your abdominal muscles are firmly clenched.

Step 4. Adjusted Limbs:
Bring your left knee up to your chest and return your right foot to the starting position to quickly switch legs.
Step 5. Make a Fast Switch:
Continue to move quickly and steadily, alternating your legs as though you were sprinting.
Step 6. Inhalation
Breathe consistently throughout the exercise, taking a breath out as you bring your knee closer to your chest and a breath in when you bring your leg back.
7. Maintain Form
Don't sag or pop your hips during the workout; instead, keep them level.
Step 8. Length of Time or Iterations:
You should perform mountain climbers for a set amount of time or repetitions; gradually raise the intensity as your fitness level rises.
Mountain climbers offer a versatile and effective way to raise heart rate while

engaging many muscle groups simultaneously, making them an excellent addition to circuit training or high-intensity interval training (HIIT).

Plank: Makes use of the core and stabilizing muscles.

Planking is a basic workout that is well known for enhancing core stability, strength, and endurance. To master the plank, you need to engage various muscle groups and appropriate form.

These are the steps to successfully complete a plank.

Step 1. Beginning Point:
Start at the hands and knees position, with your wrists exactly beneath your shoulders.
Step 2. Lean Forward:

Make a straight line from your head to your heels by extending your legs straight back with your toes on the ground.

Step 3. Activate Core:

Pull your belly button in the direction of your spine to engage your core while keeping your spine in a neutral alignment.

Step 4. Shoulder Alignment:

Keeping your shoulders back and away from your ears, contract the muscles in your upper back and shoulders.

Step 5. Hand Positioning:

Maintain a balanced weight distribution between your hands, spreading your fingers widely for support.

Step 6. Look Ahead:

To prevent tension on your neck, maintain a neutral posture by looking at the floor.

Step 7. Maintain Position:

Maintain your plank posture, making sure your body stays tight and straight.

Step 8. Inhaling:

Inhale via your nose, then exhale slowly and thoroughly through your mouth.

Step 9. Advancement:

As your strength increases, push yourself further by extending the plank's duration or attempting other variations, such as side planks or planks with lifted legs.

Planks are an effective isometric workout that works the muscles in the legs, back, and shoulders in addition to the core. For a comprehensive approach to developing stability and functional strength, include planks in your program.

A basic but effective full-body workout is jumping jacks.

Jumping jacks are a time-tested and very beneficial aerobic workout that increases heart rate, enhances coordination, and works for many muscle groups. Including jumping jacks in your exercise regimen is an excellent method to improve your general fitness. To perform a proper jumping jack, follow these steps:

Step 1. Beginning Point:

Start from a standing stance, keeping your arms by your sides and your feet together.

Step 2. Leap Ahead:

As you raise your arms aloft, jump with your feet out to the sides. An "X" should form on your body.

Step 3. Arm Layout:

Reach up toward the ceiling with your arms completely extended and your elbows slightly bent.

Step 4. Complete Extension

At the highest point of the leap, fully extend your legs and arms.

Step 5. Take Off:

Lower your arms to your sides and leap back together to revert to the beginning posture.

Step 6. Regulated Speed:

To preserve appropriate form, perform jumping jacks at a regulated and rhythmic tempo.

Step 7. Inhaling:

Throughout the workout, take natural breaths, inhaling as you jump out and exhaling as you jump in.

Step 8. Replicates:

You can incorporate jumping jacks into a dynamic warm-up or aerobic circuit, or you can perform them for a predetermined amount of repetitions to add them to your workout.

Jumping jacks are a flexible exercise that can be done at any fitness level, which makes them a great option for a rapid and effective full-body workout.

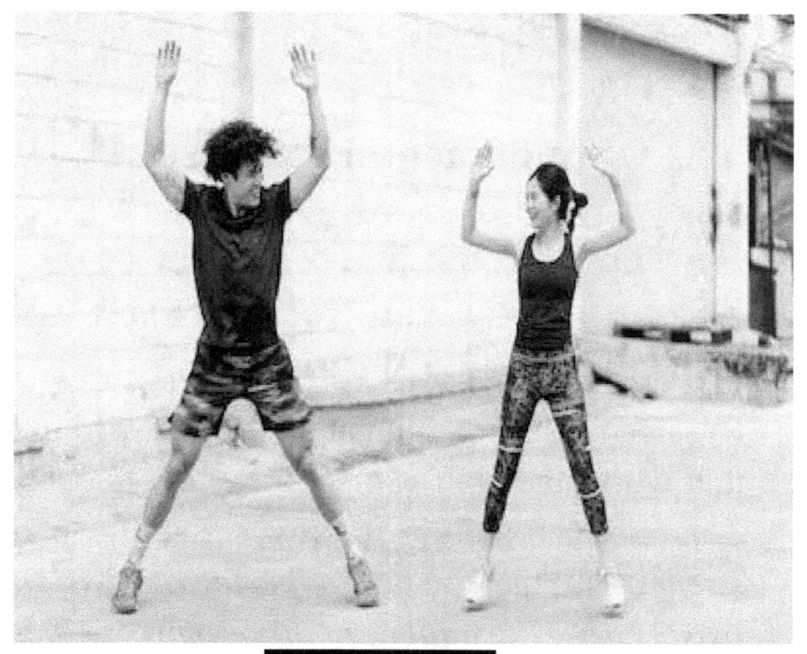
Jumping jacks

CHAPTER SEVEN

Fundamental Exercises

Russian Twists: These exercises strengthen the rotational muscles and target the obliques

Russian twists are a fun and efficient workout that works the hip flexors, core, and obliques. This circular motion improves stability and strength in the torso. ***To perform Russian twists correctly, adhere to these steps:***

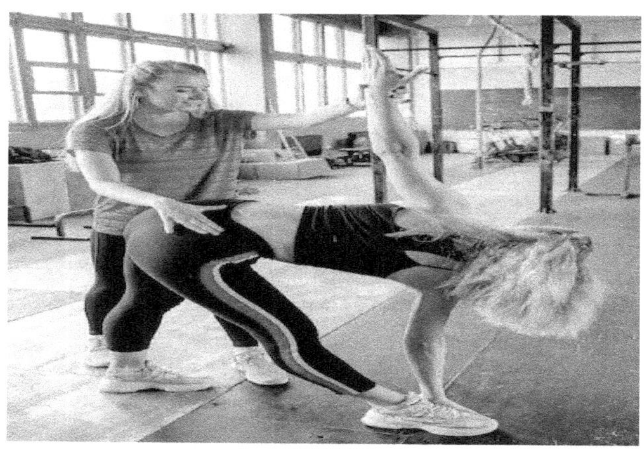

Step 1. Beginning Point:

Start by sitting on the floor with your back straight, legs bent, and feet flat.

Step 2. Recline:

Keep your core tight and strong as you slant back a little. A 45-degree angle between your body and the floor is ideal.

Step 3. Hand Positioning:

Hold a weight, medicine ball, or kettlebell at chest height, or clasp your hands together.

Step 4. Optional Leg Lifts:

Elevate your feet off the ground and balance on your sit bones for an additional challenge.

Step 5. Invert:

Turn your body to one side and move your hands or the weighted object to the floor in front of your hip. Face forward with your head and chest up.

Step Reenter the Center:

Repeat the movement in a thoughtful and controlled manner, twisting to the opposing side before returning to the center.

Step 7. Inhaling:

As you rotate to each side, release your breath and take a breath back in the center.

Step 8. Replicates:

For a thorough abdominal challenge, perform Russian twists for a set number of repetitions or include them in your core workout regimen.

Russian twists are a great complement to any core-focused exercise program because they provide strength and stability in a fun and interesting way. Depending on your degree of fitness, change the difficulty by altering the weight or the angle at which you lean.

Bicycle crunches: Increase flexibility and work the entire core.

A great abdominal workout that incorporates a dynamic, bicycle-pedaling motion and targets the rectus abdominis and obliques is the bicycle crunch. This exercise works a variety of muscle groups, which makes it a good option for developing core strength and definition. To practice bicycle crunches correctly, follow these steps:

Step 1. Beginning Point:

With your hands behind your head, elbows spread, and your legs raised off the floor to create a 90-degree angle at the hips and knees, lie on your back.

Step 2. Elbow to the Knee Across:

Take your head, feet, and shoulders off the ground.

While straightening your right leg, move your right elbow toward your left knee.

Step 3. Pedaling a bike:

While straightening your left leg, pedal by raising your left elbow to your right knee. Maintain this alternate gait of pedaling a bicycle.

Step 4. Engage Core:

Throughout the exercise, keep your lower back pressed into the floor by engaging your core.

Step 5. Inhaling:

Breathe in as you switch sides, then exhale as you spin and bring your elbow to the other knee.

Step 6. Regulated Speed:

Cycle crunches should be performed at a slow, steady tempo with an emphasis on quality rather than quantity.

Step 7. Replicates:

Bike crunches are a great addition to any ab training regimen; try to complete a set number of reps to properly challenge and improve your core.

Bike crunches are a strenuous and dynamic abdominal exercise that will help you develop a toned and powerful stomach. Include them in your program.For best results, adjust the difficulty to your current level of fitness and advance gradually.

CHAPTER EIGHT

Monitoring Development

Any fitness journey must include tracking your progress because it gives you important insights into your accomplishments and keeps you motivated. Here are some essential pointers for efficiently monitoring your progress:

- **Make definite goals:**

Establish *SMART* goals, which stand for specified, measurable, achievable, relevant, and time-bound. Whether the goal is increased endurance, strength development, or weight loss, setting specific goals makes it easier to monitor your progress.

- **Employ Measurements**

Note baseline data such as body weight, measurements, and percentage of body fat. Review these indicators on a regular basis to keep an eye out for changes and modify your strategy as necessary.

- **Record Your Workouts:**

Keep a thorough exercise journal that details the exercises, sets, repetitions, and weights used. This enables you to monitor your strength improvements, spot trends, and modify your training regimen intelligently.

- **Capture Fitness Evaluations:**

Use performance-based tests, such as timed runs, maximum push-ups, or flexibility evaluations, to periodically gauge your level of fitness. These standards offer concrete indicators of advancement.

- **Capture Images of Progress:**

Progress images that are visually documented can be a very effective motivator. Take pictures from different perspectives on a regular basis to track physical changes over time.

- **Make Use of Fitness Apps**

Numerous fitness applications come with options for tracking overall progress, nutrition, and activities. Charts and graphs are frequently used in these apps to show achievements and trends.

- **Take Note of Your Body:**

Observe your body's sensations and functions. Qualitative markers of success include improved sleep, elevated mood, and increased energy levels.

- **Honor Significant Occasions:**

Celebrate and give recognition to both minor and major accomplishments. Acknowledging progress makes it easier to stay motivated and have a good outlook.

- **Modify and Turn:**

Adopt a flexible strategy. Never be afraid to make changes to your exercise regimen, diet, or overall approach based on your progress statistics if something isn't working.

- **Key to Consistency:**

Development requires time. Continue to put in constant work, and have faith in the process. The significance of your dedication to long-term health and fitness is reinforced by regular tracking.

Maintaining focus, adjusting to shifts, and attaining long-lasting outcomes in your fitness journey all depend on you keeping a regular assessment and tracking of your progress. Consistent tracking is an important success tool, regardless of whether you decide to employ measures, technology, or in-person evaluations.

Defining Quantifiable Objectives

Establishing quantifiable objectives is essential to monitoring your progress and maintaining motivation while you pursue fitness. **The following are crucial actions to set quantifiable goals:**

- **Be Particular:**

Clearly state your objective. Rather than settling for a general goal like **"lose weight,"** **choose a specific goal like "lose 10 pounds."**

- **Apply Numbers:**

Include monetary values in your objectives. This could be the amount of weight to lift, the distance to run, or the number of pounds to drop.

- **Put it in Reach:**

Make sure your objective is reachable in the allotted time. Unattainable objectives could cause frustration.

- **Design a Timetable:**

Give yourself a deadline to finish the task at hand. This keeps you focused and instills a sense of urgency.

- **To put it simply:**

If your objective is big, divide it up into more attainable, smaller goals. Reaching these tiny objectives helps you stay motivated.

- **Use Verbs of Action:**

Use language that will help you achieve your aim. Say **"finish a 5k run in 8 weeks"** as an example, rather than **"get in shape."**

- **Including Frequency:**

Indicate how frequently you plan to carry out the tasks necessary to reach your objective. Suppose you were to **"exercise for 30 minutes, five times a week."**

- **Establish Accountability**

Tell a friend or exercise partner about your objectives so they can encourage you and keep you responsible.

- **Monitor Development:**

Decide on your progress measurement strategy. Quantifiable measures are crucial for tracking calories, documenting exercise data, and monitoring body measurements.

- **Honor accomplishments:**

When you accomplish milestones, plan modest celebrations. Acknowledging successes encourages positive conduct.

- **A Measurable Goal Example Would Be:**

In particular, "Lose 10 pounds."

Measurable: Monitor your development and weigh yourself frequently.

Realistic: Aiming for a weekly weight loss of one to two pounds.

Set a deadline for yourself: "Lose 10 pounds in the next 8 weeks."

The suggestion is to "exercise for 30 minutes, five times a week."

Simplify it to: "Achieve a weight loss of 2 pounds during the initial 2 weeks, 3 pounds during the subsequent 3 weeks, and 5 pounds during the last 3 weeks."

By giving yourself a clear road map for your fitness journey, quantifiable goals help you stay accountable, inspired, and focused.

Modifying The Plan Based On Results

A key component of attaining long-term success is modifying your exercise program in response to your outcomes. Taking regular stock of your progress enables you to make calculated changes to maximize your strategy. If you're exceeding your objectives, think about stepping up your effort or establishing new benchmarks to push yourself even more.

Conversely, if the pace of advancement is less than anticipated, reconsider the efficacy of your plan. This could entail modifying your exercise regimen, modifying your diet, or reassessing your recuperation techniques. Adaptability and attentiveness to your body's signals are essential; a dynamic exercise regimen that changes based on your performance guarantees ongoing inspiration and progress. Adapting the plan in response to your fitness goals is a wise and flexible approach, not a sign of failure.

It's also critical to pay attention to how your body reacts to different workouts or food choices. It's critical to change course and look into alternatives if a certain exercise regimen isn't working out or if a certain diet isn't producing the desired effects. This flexibility promotes a more pleasurable and long-lasting journey towards fitness.

Keeping a regular eye on your energy levels, sleep quality, and general well-being might yield insightful information for improvements. Speaking with dietitians or fitness experts can provide knowledgeable advice and guarantee that your approach is in line with your changing objectives. Recall that being adaptable in your approach shows a dedication to ongoing improvement rather than a sign of weakness, making the pursuit of ideal health and fitness a dynamic and unique experience.

The Value Of Seeking Advice From Fitness experts

Getting advice from fitness experts is essential to making the most of your path toward wellness and health. These professionals offer specific expertise, real-world experience, and tailored advice to guarantee that you safely and effectively meet your fitness objectives.

Whether your goal is increased general fitness, weight loss, or strength gain, fitness experts like personal trainers can create customized exercise plans that meet your unique goals. They guarantee ideal muscle engagement and assist in preventing injuries by giving appropriate guidance on training routines.

Dietitians, or nutritionists, who are frequently associated with the fitness industry, provide vital advice on creating a sustainable and well-balanced diet. They can help with meal planning, handle dietary restrictions, and teach you about the nutritional aspects of providing your body with the fuel it needs to function at its best.

Fitness experts can also act as accountability partners and motivators to help you stick to your program. They monitor your development, make the required corrections, and acknowledge your successes. The knowledge and skills of these experts improve the efficacy and security of your fitness journey, regardless of your level of experience, making consultation a prudent investment in your long-term health.

Fitness experts are also essential in developing a regimented and advanced training program. They can modify exercises to take into account any restrictions or current health issues, making sure your fitness regimen is safe and challenging. This individualized care makes the experience more efficient and pleasurable, avoiding monotony and encouraging sticking to your exercise regimen.

For people who are new to exercising, seeking advice from fitness experts is especially important. They impart knowledge on basic concepts, appropriate forms, and the science underlying different training modalities. People are better equipped to make decisions regarding their health thanks to this knowledge.

Fitness experts frequently act as motivators in the field of mental health, providing support and encouragement during trying times. Their knowledge goes beyond the tangible and includes techniques for stress reduction, better sleep, and cultivating an optimistic outlook.

Consulting with experts guarantees that you stay up to date on the most recent industry practices as the fitness environment is always changing due to new research and trends. This continuing education promotes a comprehensive approach to health by giving you the skills to manage the complexity of wellness and fitness. In summary, working with fitness experts enhances your fitness journey and makes it more meaningful, sustainable, and successful.

CONCLUSION

The journey towards adopting a more active and health-conscious lifestyle is characterized by personal development, perseverance, and the transforming influence of self-control. These activities are the compass pointing us in the direction of our best selves when we consider how important it is to set quantifiable goals, monitor our progress, and modify our plans in response to outcomes.

Fitness is dynamic, meaning it takes mental toughness in addition to physical work. We provide ourselves a road map when we establish specific, attainable goals, which transform ambitions into real objectives. Keeping a regular progress log helps us stay motivated by highlighting small wins that we may otherwise miss. Adapting our strategies in response to outcomes is proof of our dedication to ongoing progress rather than a sign

of failure.

Consulting with fitness experts gives this trip an extra degree of knowledge and assistance. Their advice—whether it's in the form of customized exercise plans, dietary recommendations, or moral support—improves the efficacy and durability of our endeavors. They play a part in our quest for well-being that goes beyond simple guidance.

The main lesson is to be flexible as we traverse the varied terrain of fitness. Being able to change course, evaluate our strategy, and recalibrate it is a strength in and of itself. Being fit is a process that never ends; each step we take shows how committed we are to our health and development.

Essentially, the end of the fitness journey is not a point of completion but rather an epiphany—that is, the awareness that maintaining our health is a lifetime endeavor. By establishing objectives, monitoring advancement, modifying strategies, and pursuing direction, we set out on a life-changing journey that surpasses the tangible, enhancing all aspects of our existence. Accept the path, enjoy the obstacles, and bask in the deep effects of a comprehensive commitment to a more vibrant and healthy existence.